FRIENDSHIP TEA

By
Sharon O. Maida

Lillian Rankel

Illustrated by

Danijela Popovic

Authors' Note

This book has been written for the blind and low-vision children of Africa, and their families and friends. It will be introduced at St. Joseph's Kiomiti School for the Blind in Gesusu, Kenya where young children and their families are being brought together to learn and share ideas about independence and safety and to meet the educational aspirations of the children.

Children who live close to the school will live in their homes while others will have the opportunity to reside at two recently-built dormitories. This book is the first in a series of 4 books which chronicle different situations that blind and low vision children face. Our wish is that these books will bring acceptance, independence, happiness and empowerment to blind and low vision children throughout Africa and the rest of the world!!

©2017 by The James and Sharon Maida Foundation

All Rights Reserved

ISBN-13:978-1542993913 ISBN-10:1542993911

Book preparation, formatting and submission by Bearly Tolerable Publications.

The verdana 16 pt. font used in this book is the recommended font for the visually impaired.

The line spacing is set at 1.5, as recommended by the American Foundation for the Blind.

Many thanks to:

William Bentrim for his diligent guidance.

To the many students, with and without vision, who have taught us countless lessons throughout our careers in education.

To each of our own children who are constant reminders of why happiness and independence for ALL children is paramount!

After I put on my dress and sweater, my Mother and I eat a quick breakfast of tea and cooked corn with milk. Our goat gives us milk every day.

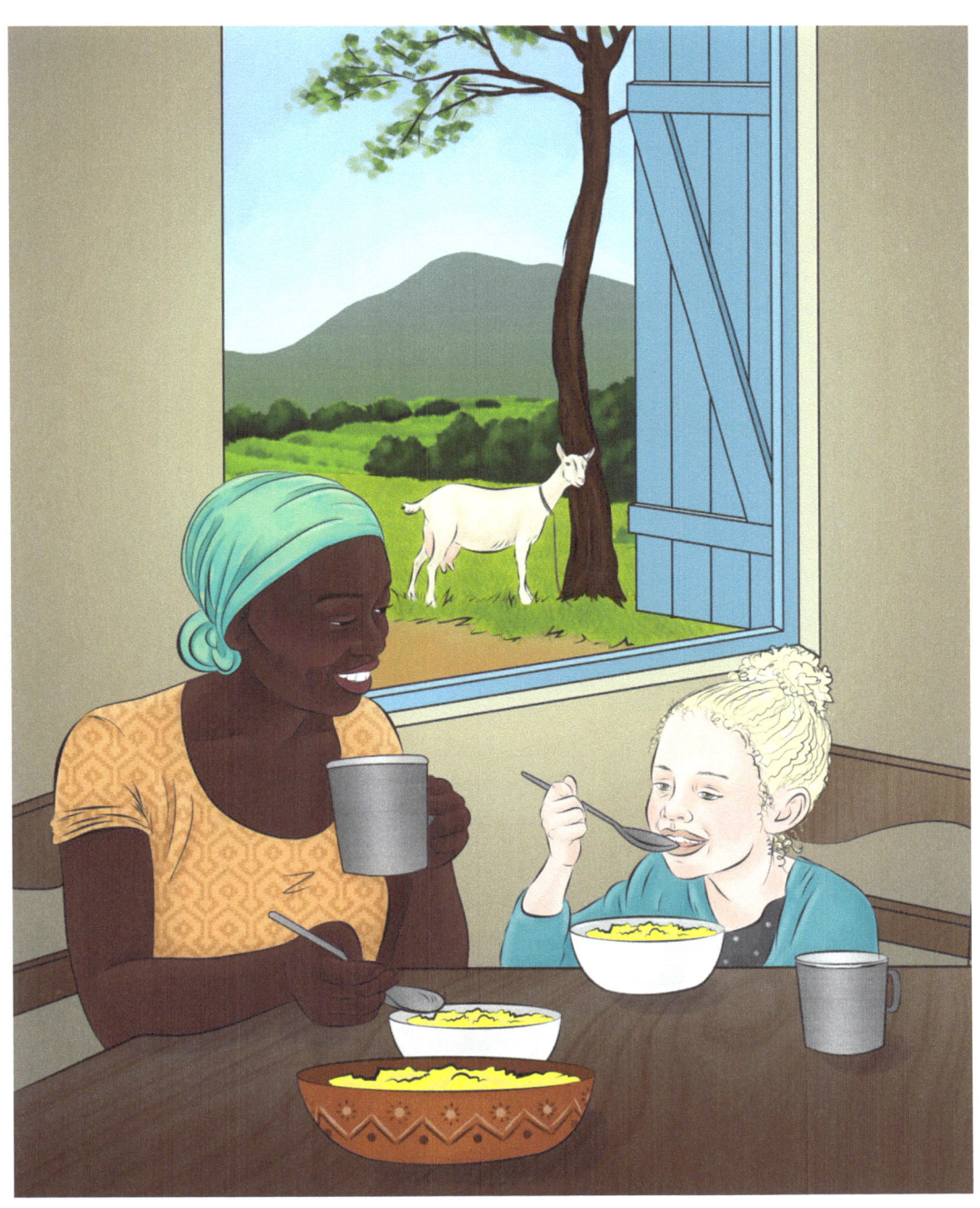

I love to get up early before the sun is too bright! We then go behind our house to our large plot and pick tea. I have a small basket across my shoulder for the collected leaves.

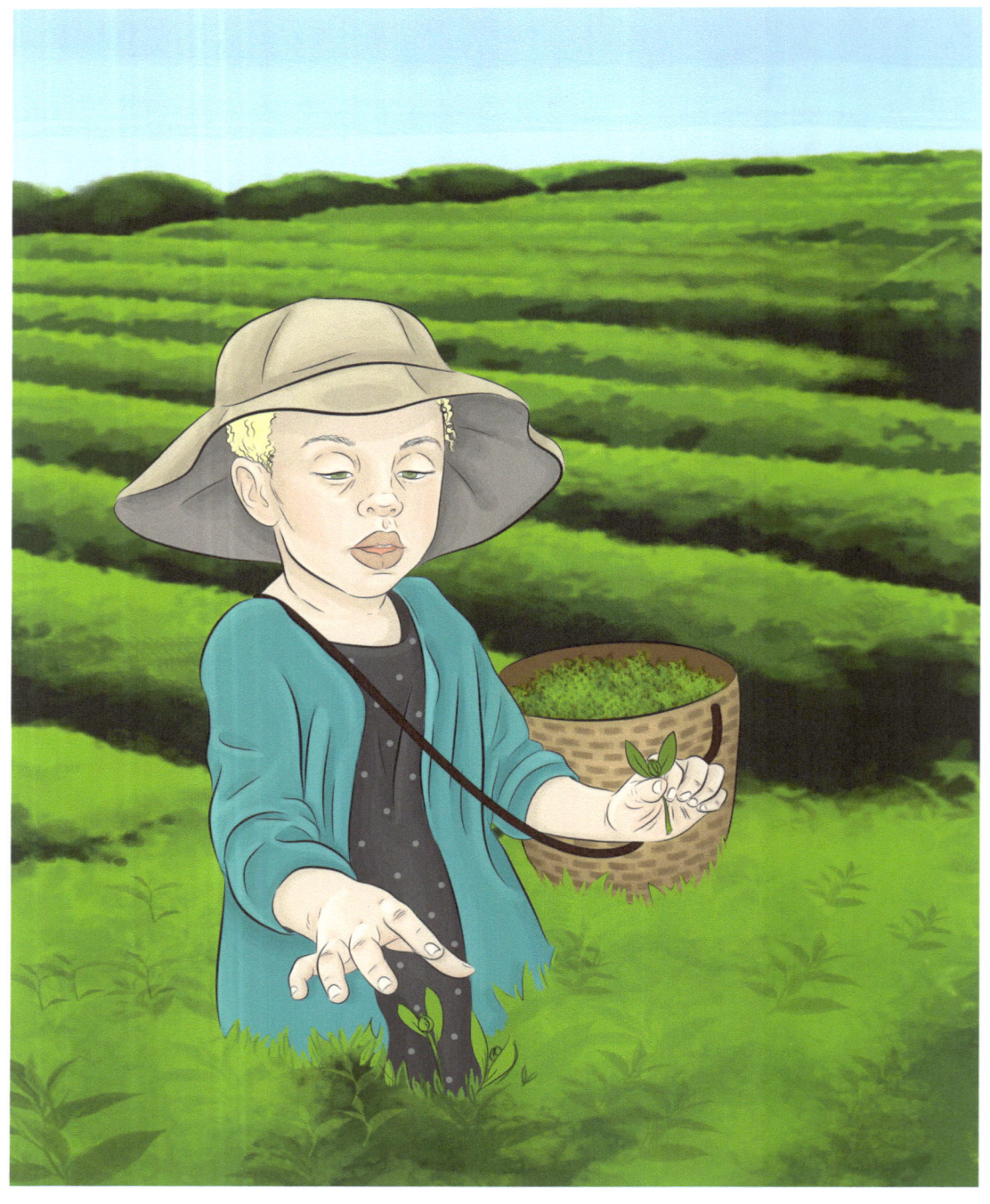

"Two leaves and a bud", I keep saying to myself so that I pick the right part from the tea bushes.

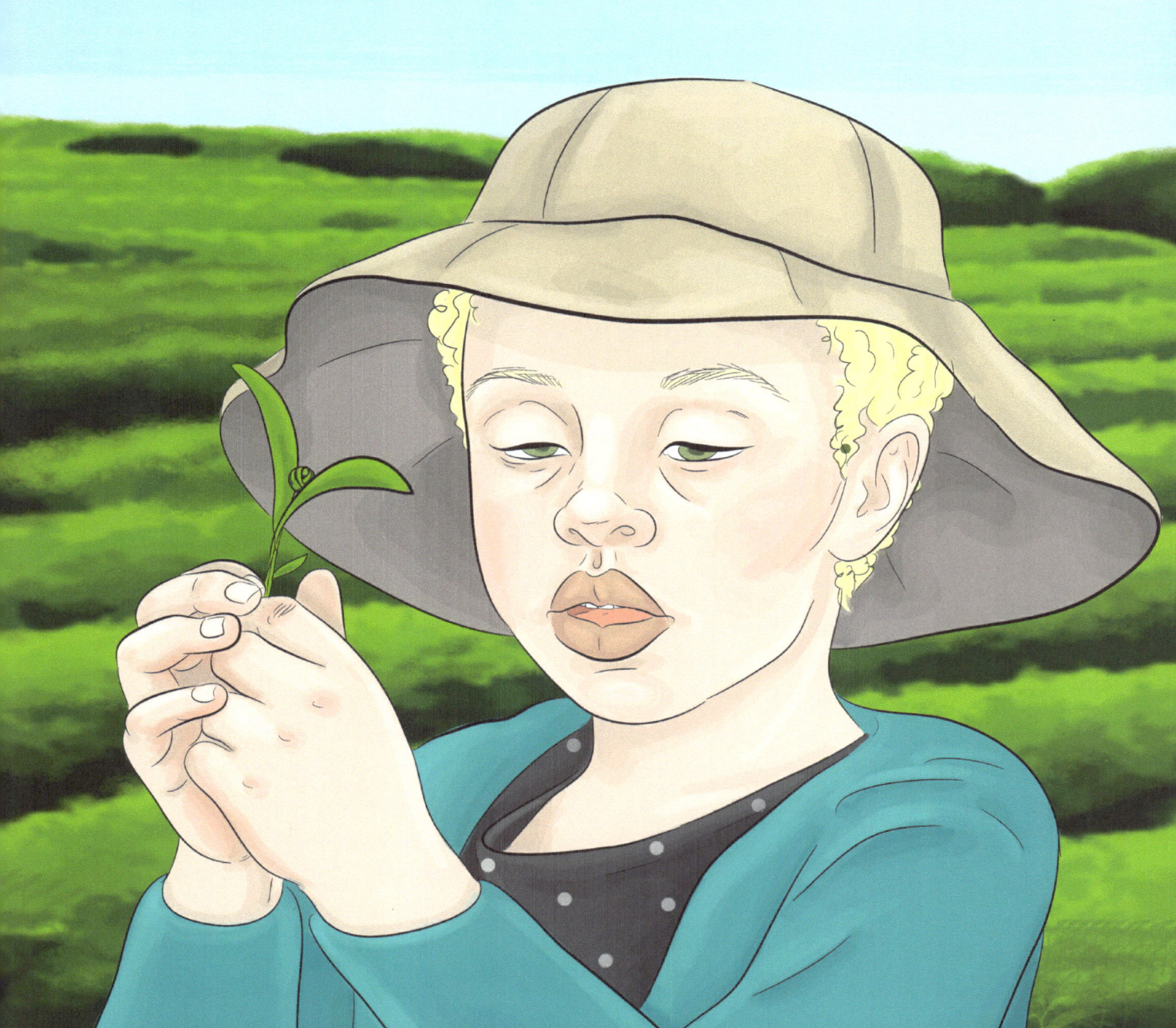

4

After an hour, my small basket is full of leaves. I call to Mother that my basket is full and she comes over to look at my leaves.

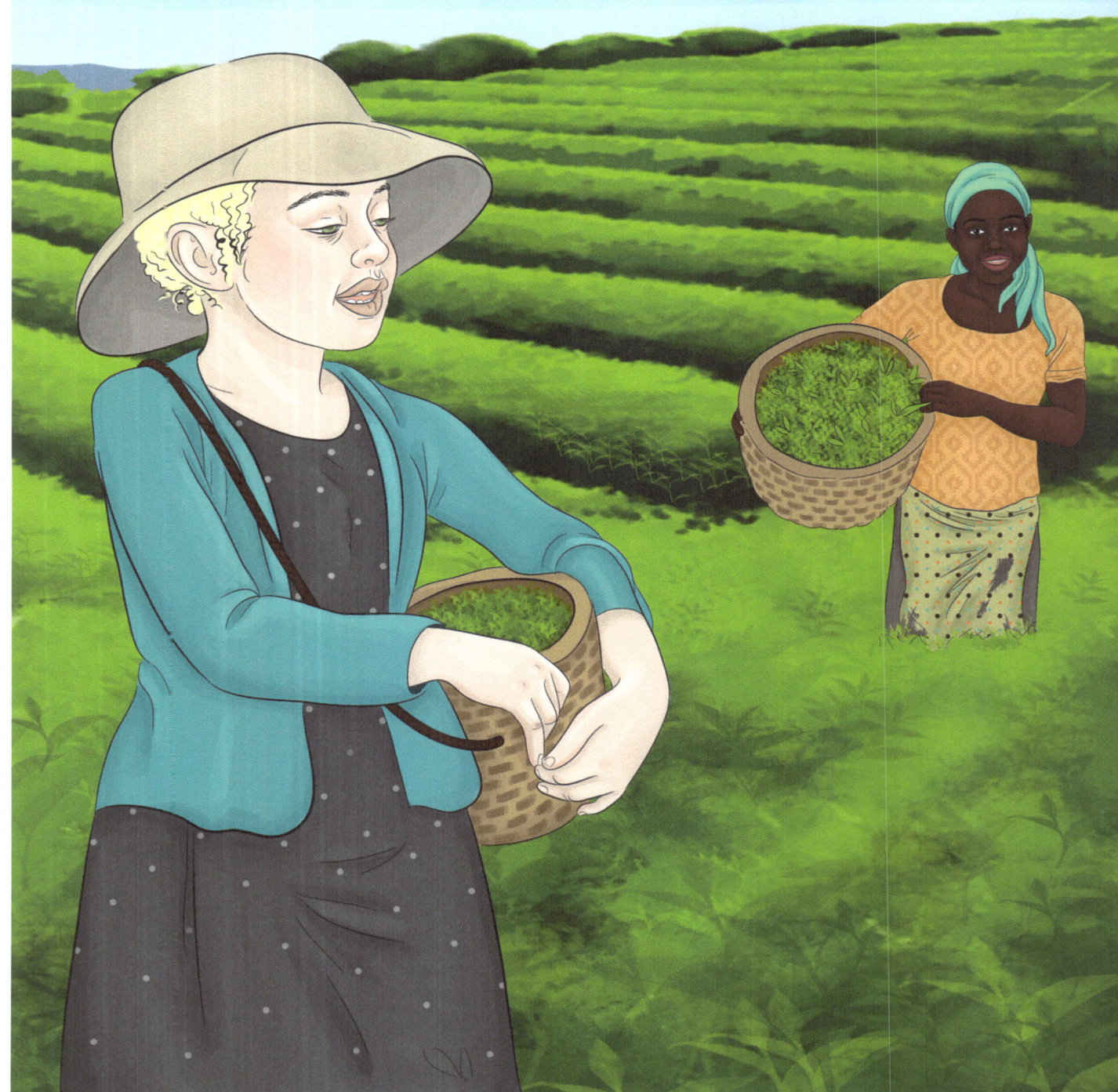

Mother says, "Rose, you are such a good tea picker gathering two leaves and a bud". She adds my leaves to her basket and now her basket is full of the dark green leaves.

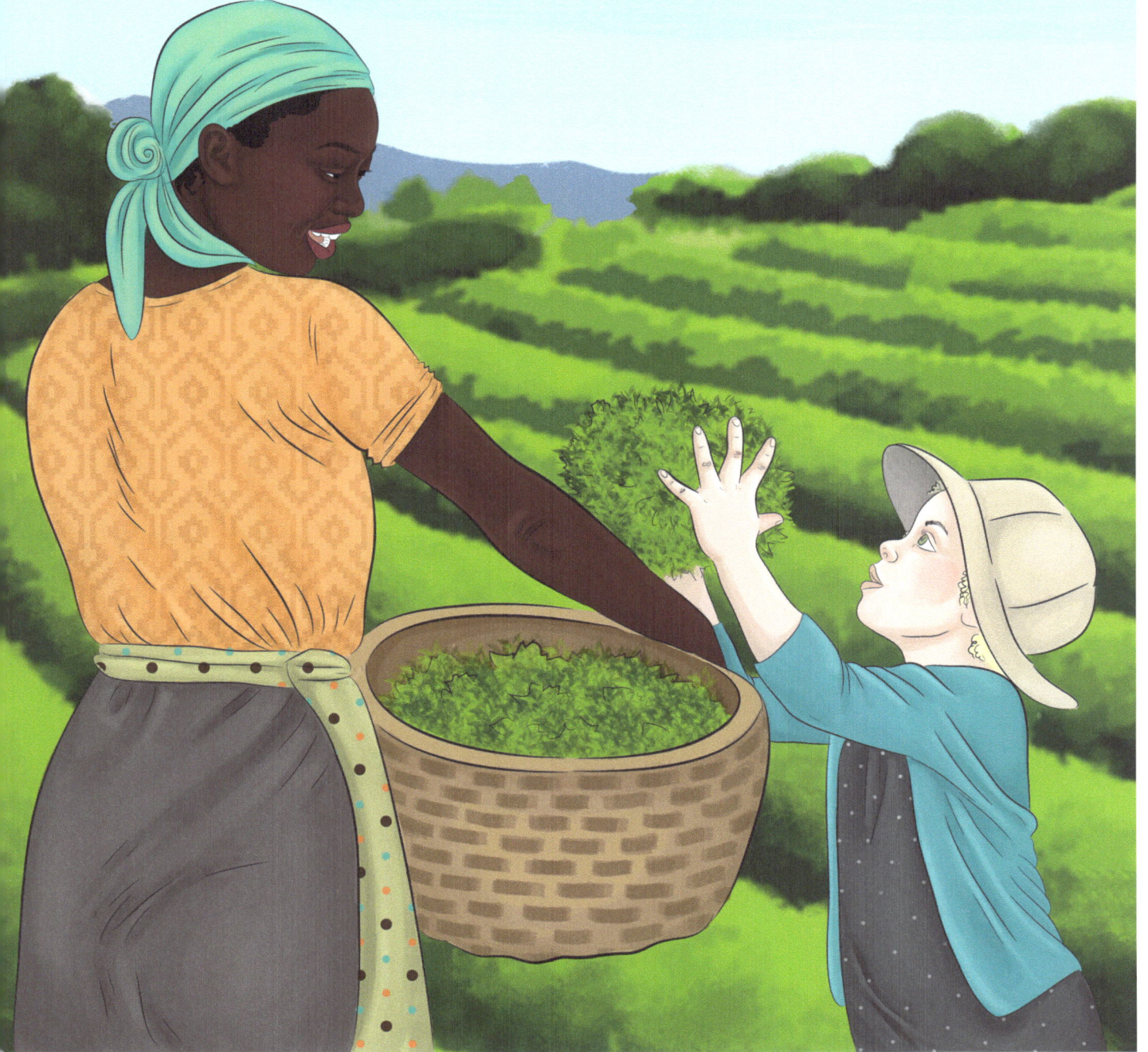

6

We are very hot from collecting the tea in the strong sunlight, so we go back to the house and wash our faces and hands before walking to the tea buying center with our basket of tea.

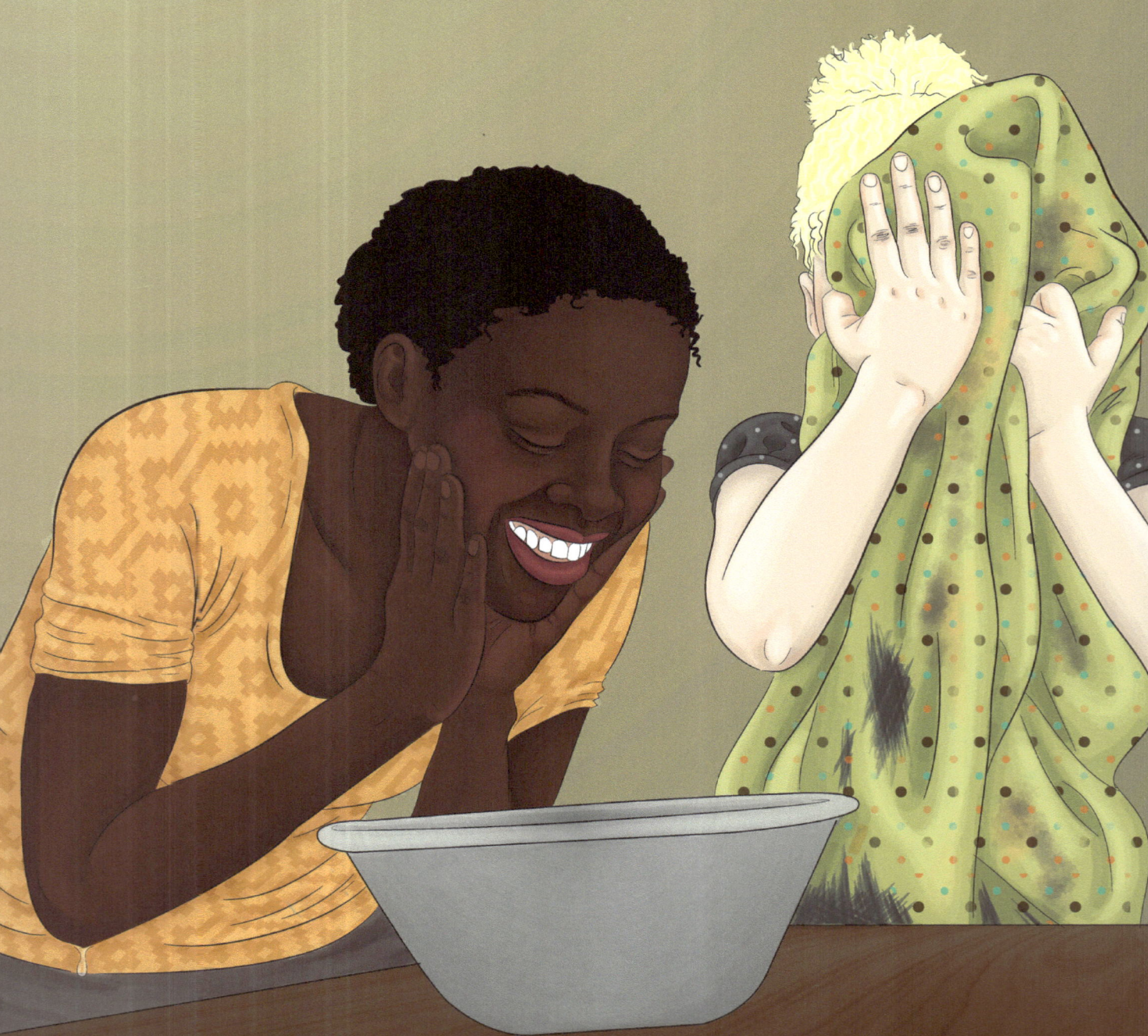

Mother holds my hand when we walk. I am a six-year-old albino girl and cannot see distant things very well. Bright sunlight hurts my eyes.

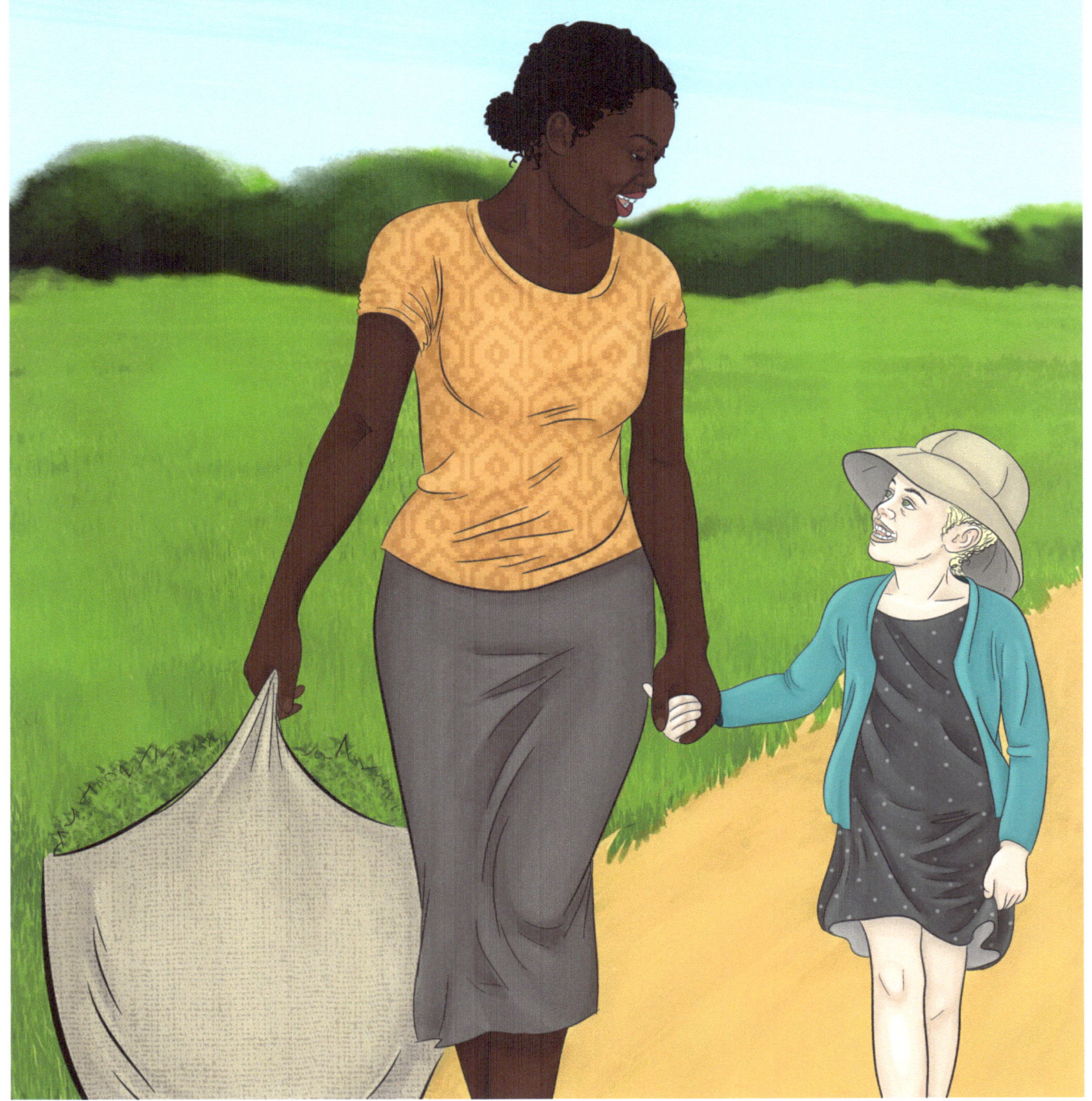

I always wear a large hat to keep the sun off my face and a long sleeved dress. My skin is white and my hair is yellow, so I can get sunburned quickly in the strong Kenyan sun.

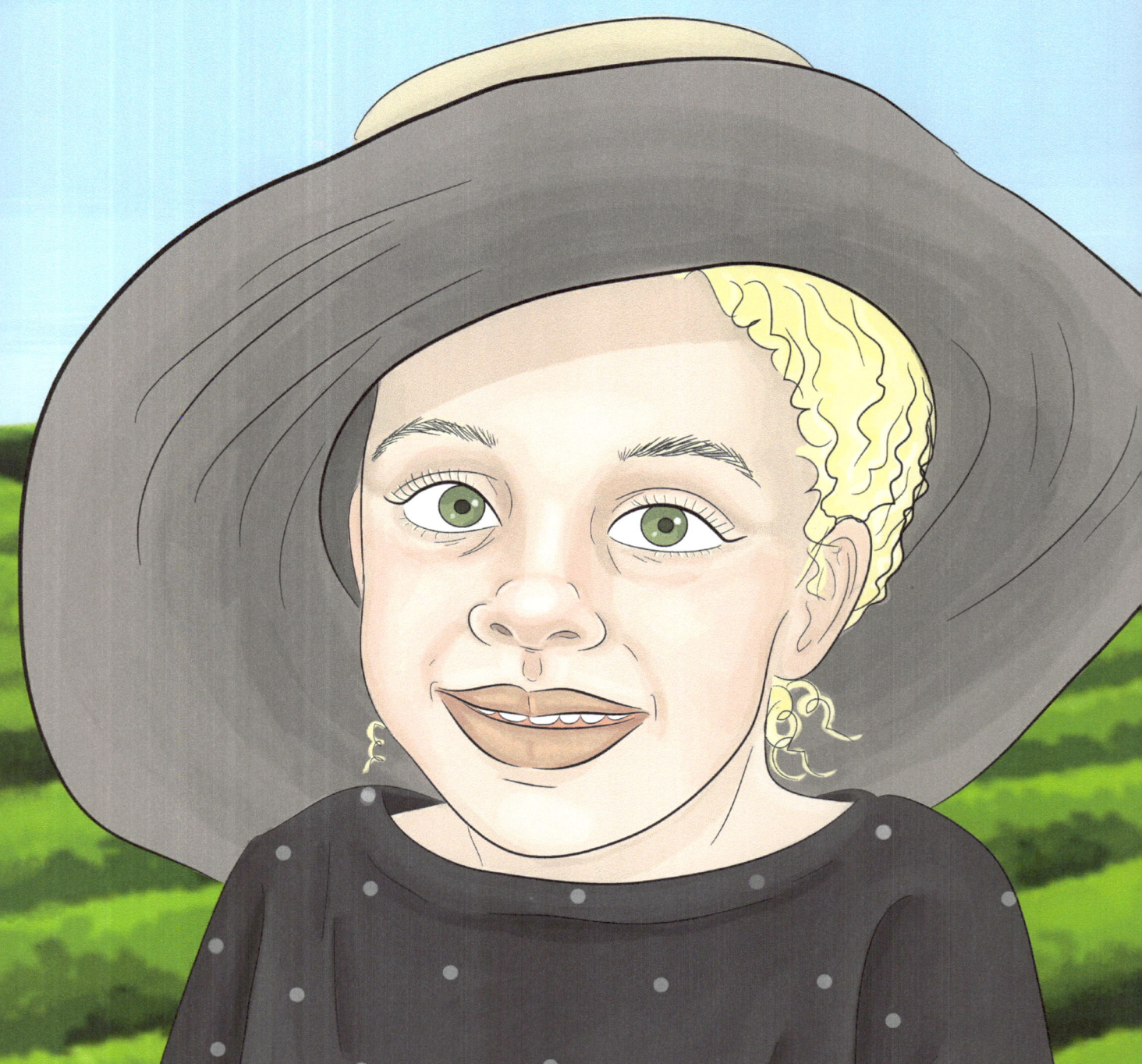

My Mother's skin is dark brown but I was born with white skin. Mother tells me that I, too, am one of God's children. All God's children come in many different colors.

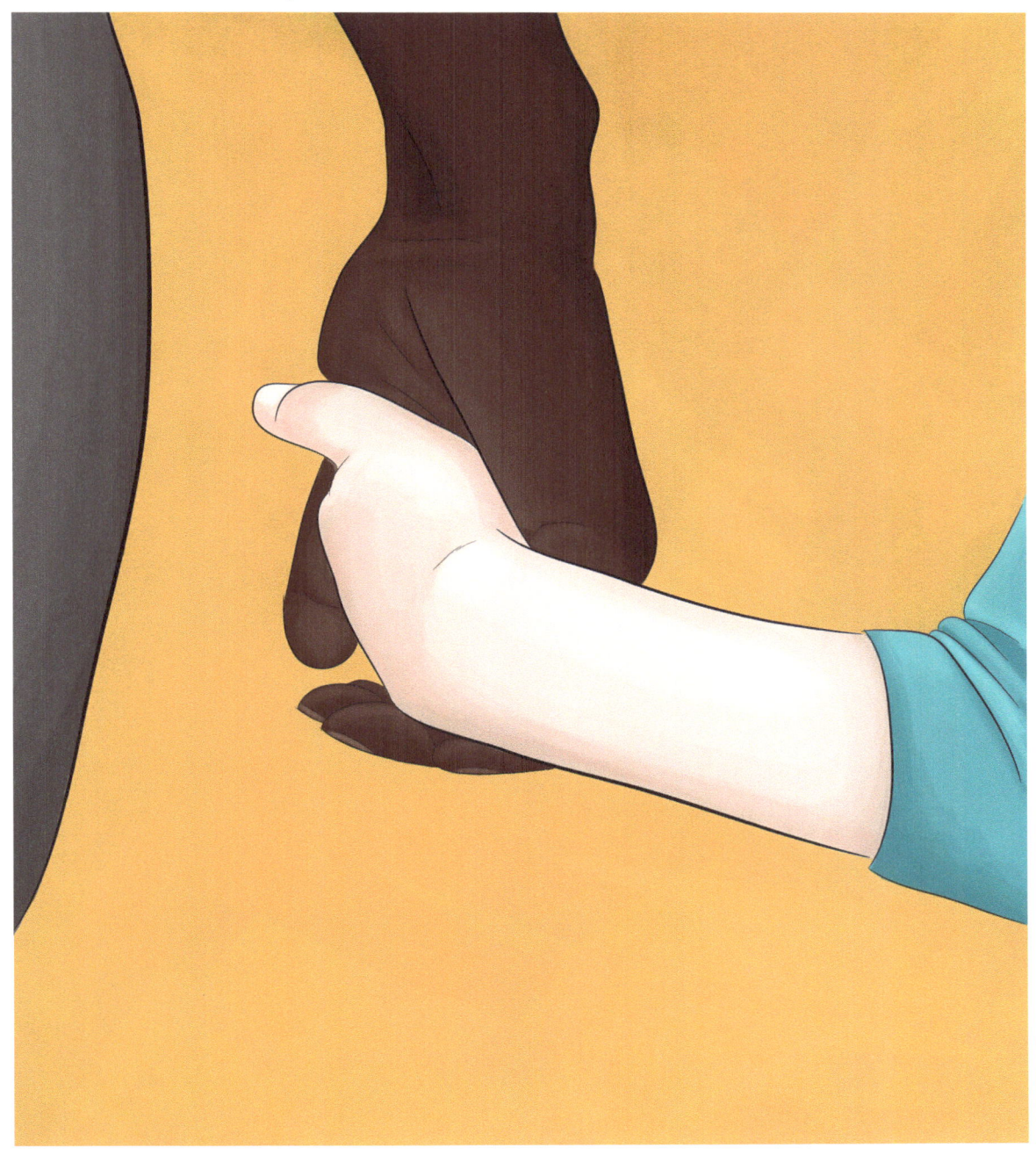

I like going to the tea buying center once a week because I always see my friend Margaret there with her mother, who is also selling her freshly picked tea leaves.

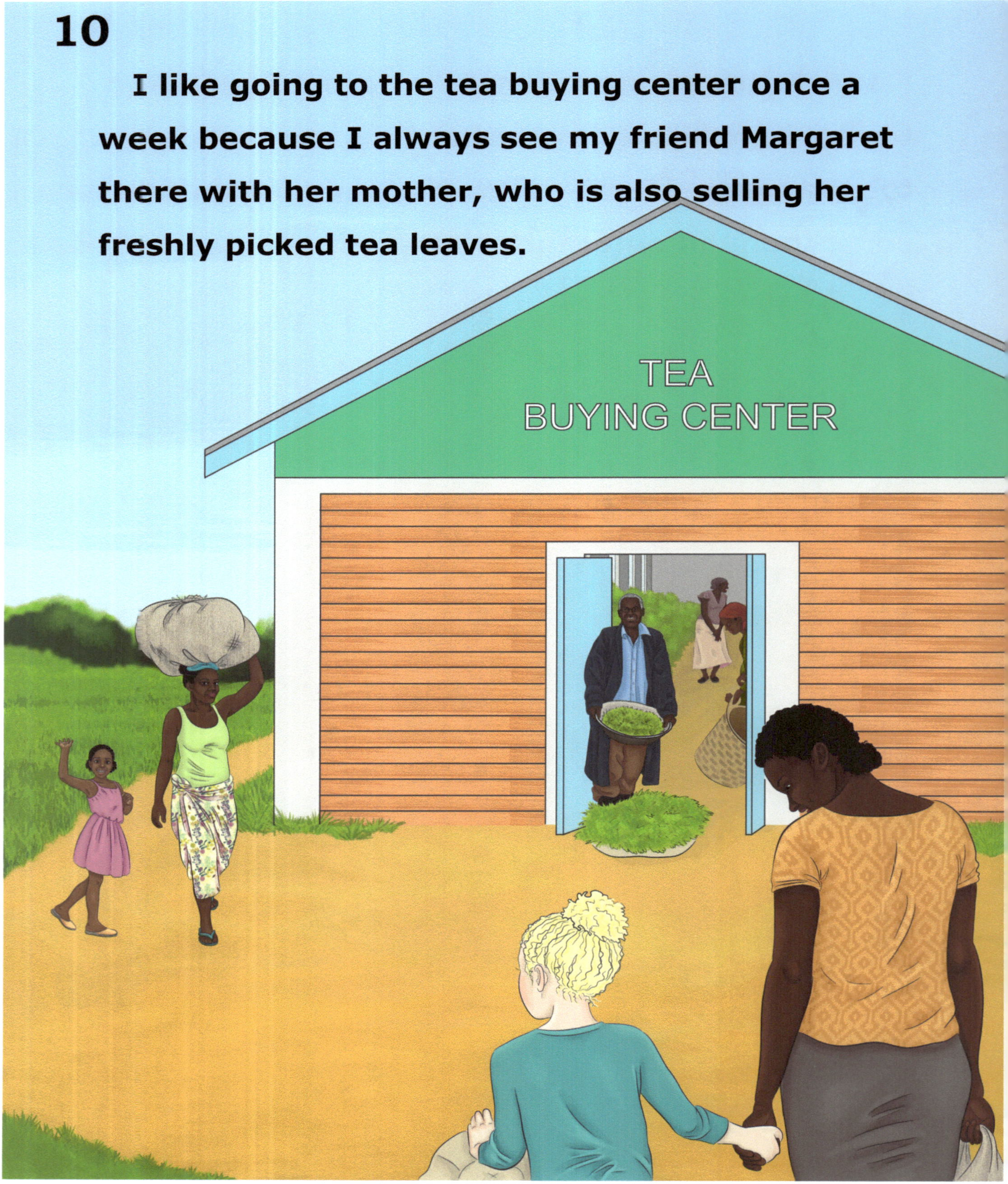

While the women are waiting in line to weigh and sell the tea, Margaret and I go out of the side door.   We look for a shady spot to sit because I try to stay out of the sun as much as possible.

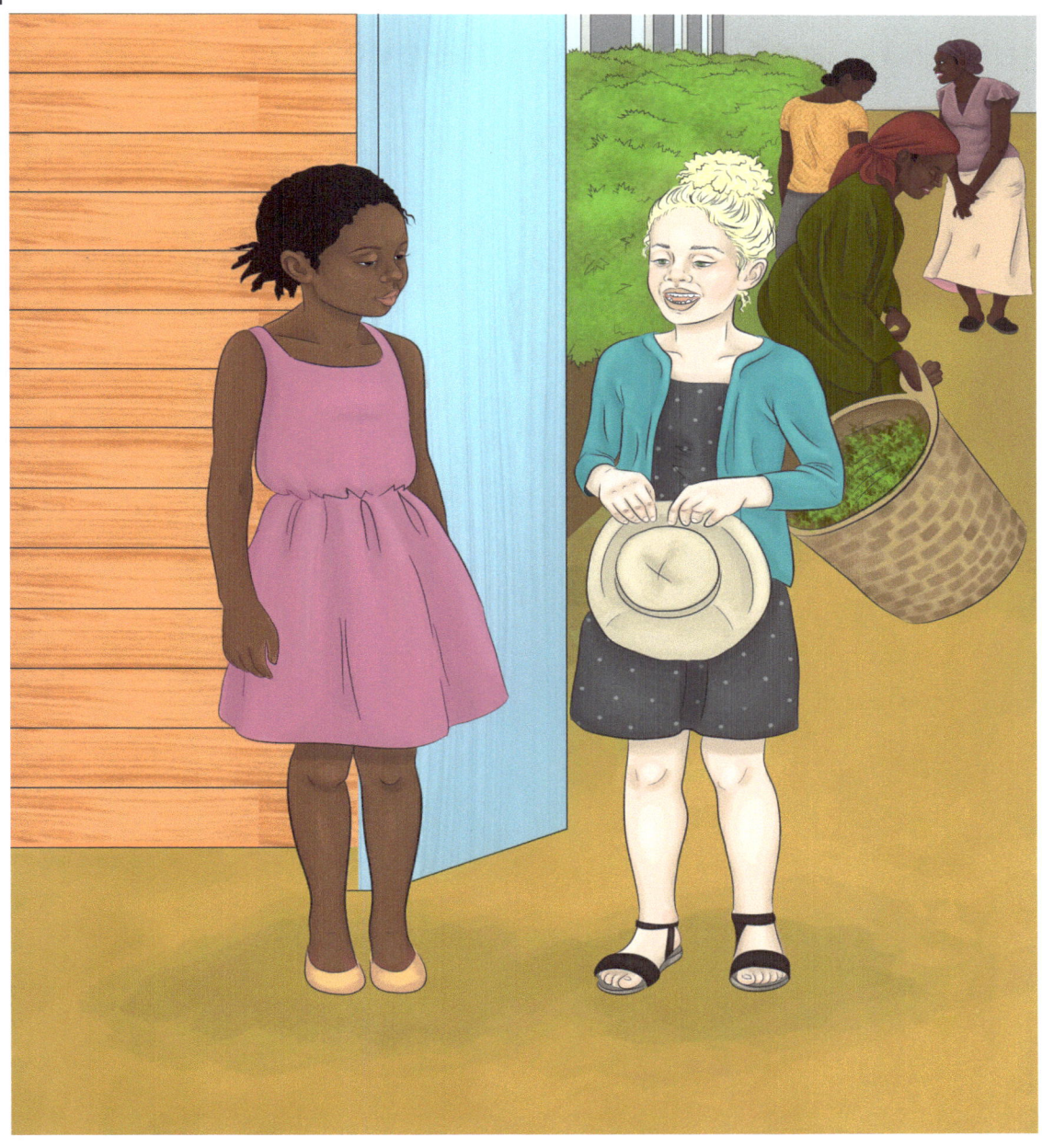

Margaret has a special treat that we can share today and she takes a very large green avocado out of her pocket. She sits on the grass and carefully peels off the skin and we take turns taking bites out of the avocado.

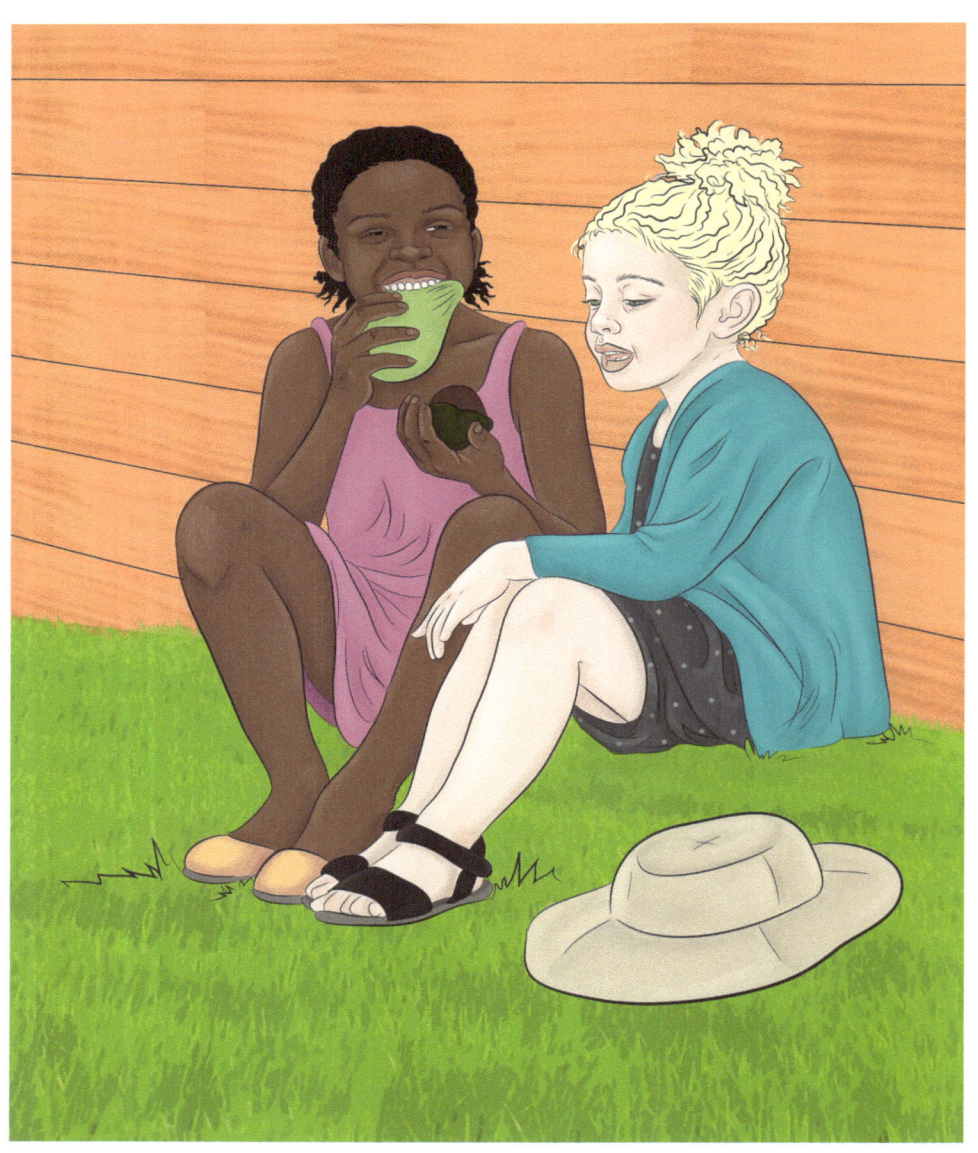

This avocado grew on the tree near her house. Soon all that is left of the avocado is the large, hard center pit. Margaret suggests that I take the avocado pit home and grow an avocado tree in our garden.

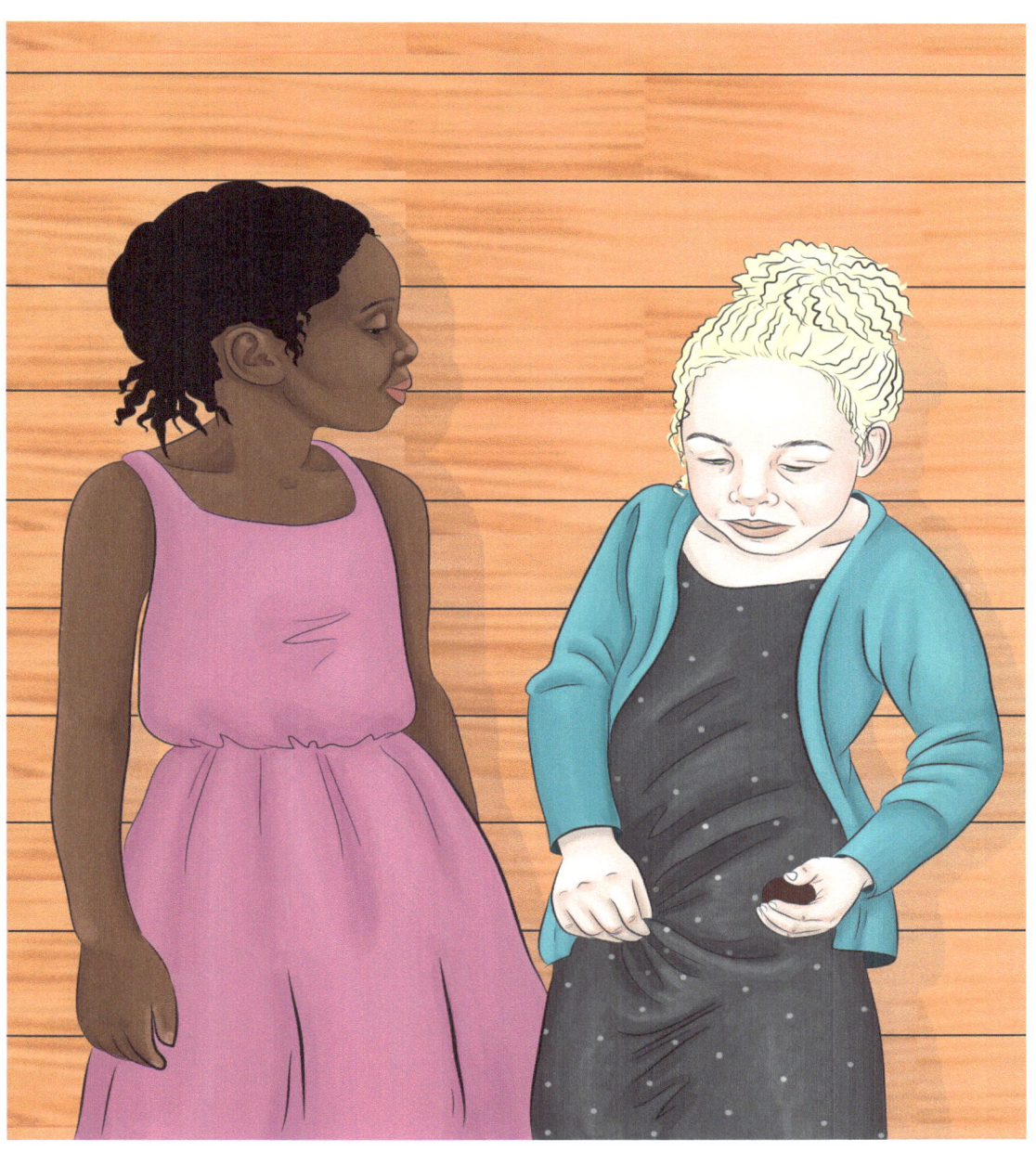

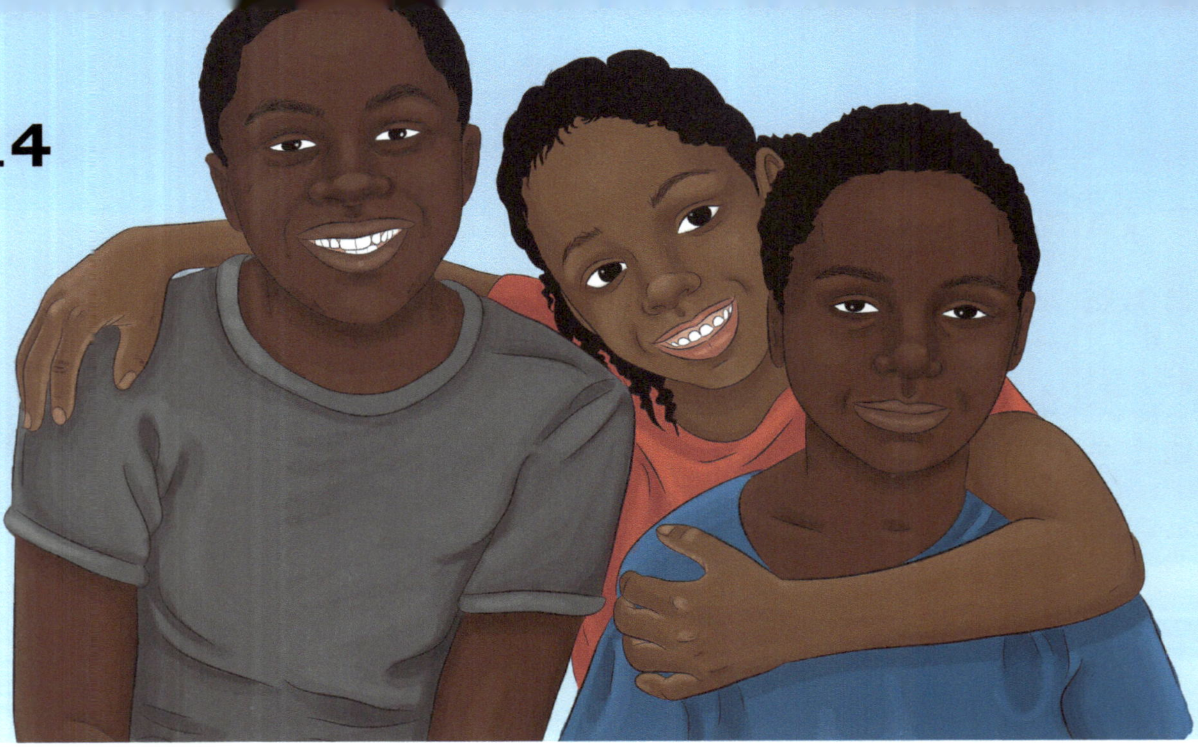

We sit on the ground and talk about our lives and our families. Both Margaret and I have two older brothers who go to school every day.

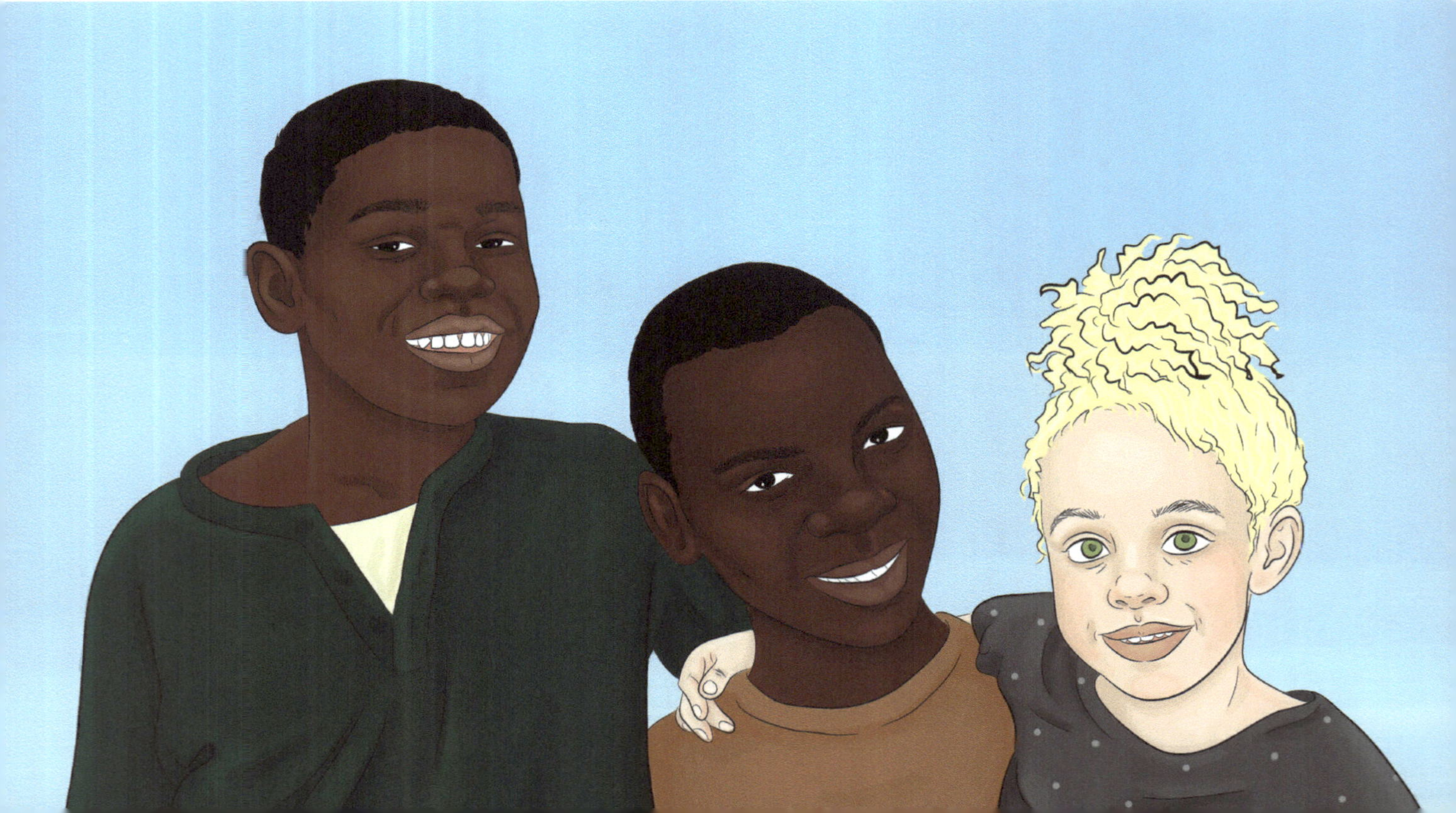

Margaret and I are excited to start school in January. Margaret will go to a nearby school with her two brothers. Margaret's mother is saving money from selling tea to buy her a dark blue uniform for school.

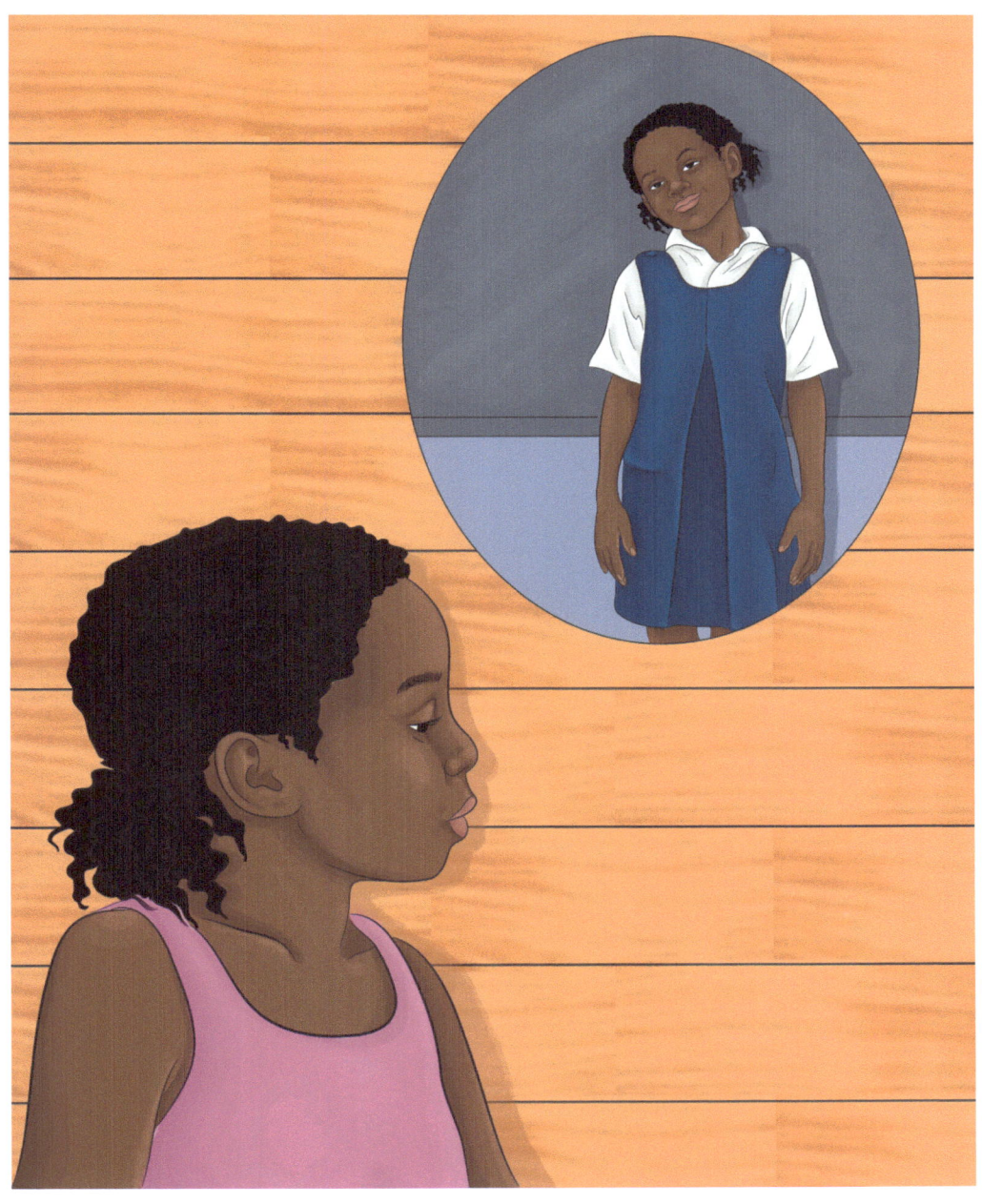

I will be going to a boarding school for children who are blind or visually impaired. The school is far away so I will live in the dormitory with other girls and learn there.

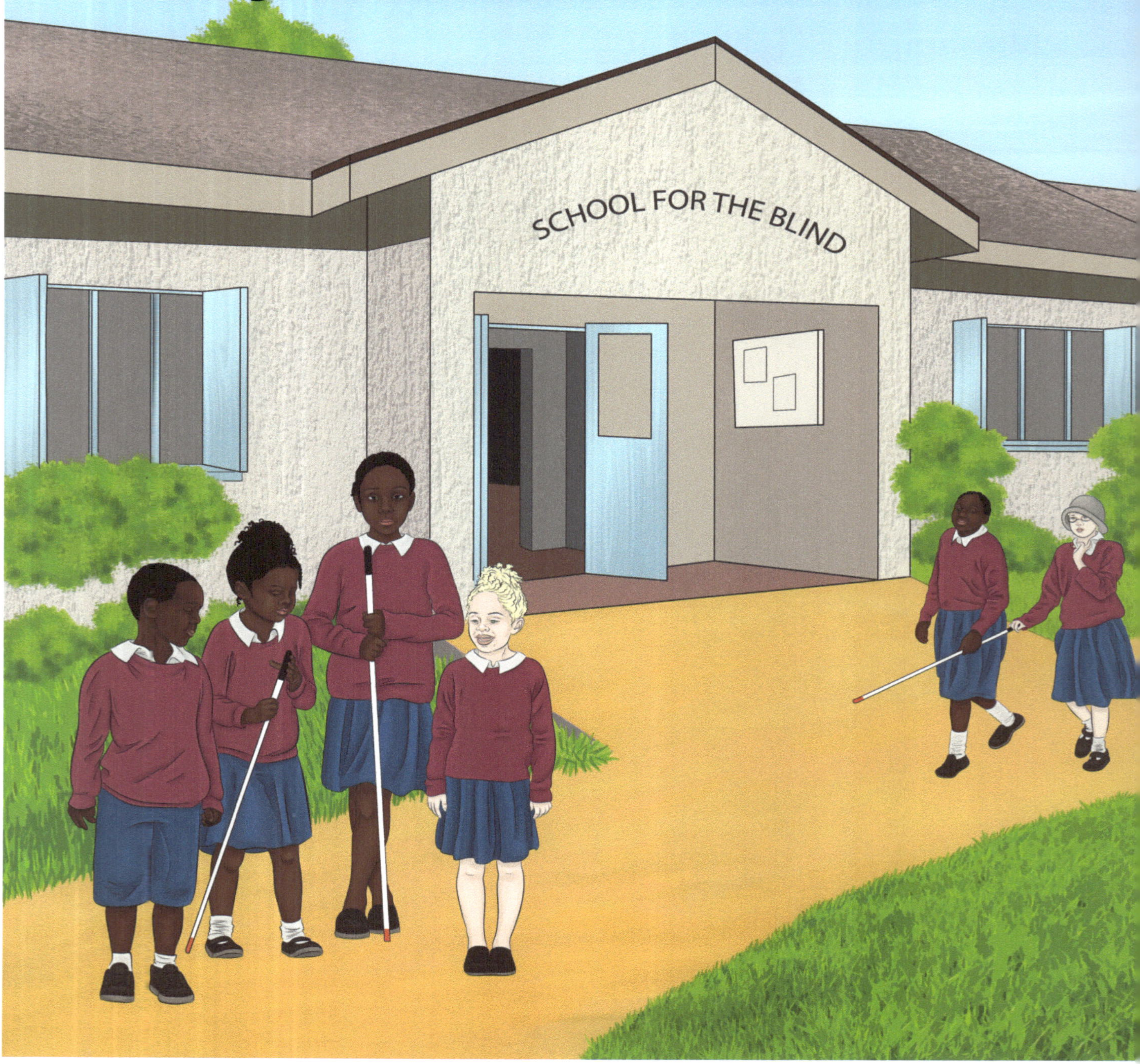

Classes are seven days a week at my school and I will be able to come home during school breaks. My mother is saving money to buy me a mattress and blanket to use at the school.

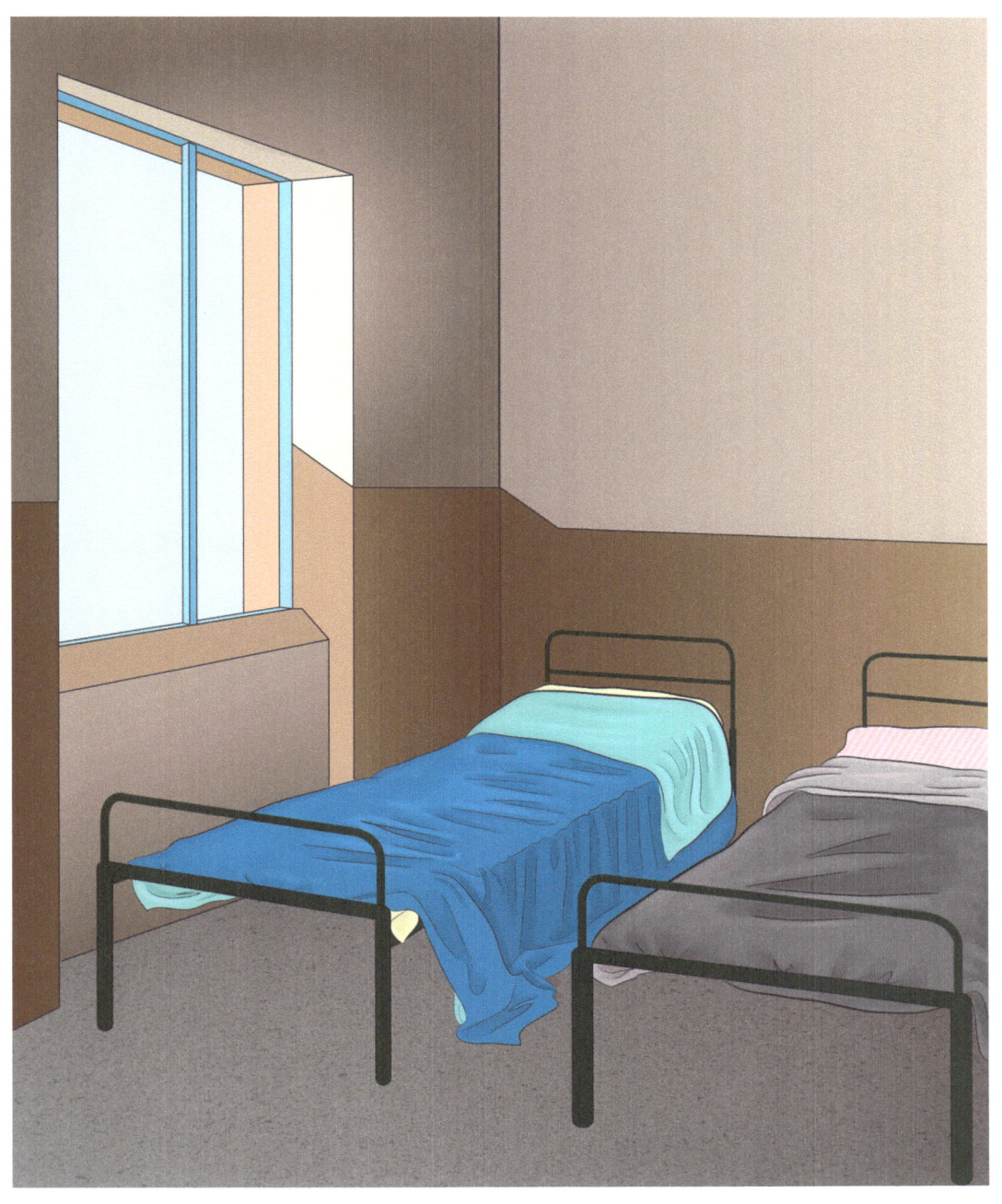

There will be many other albino children at the school and no one will stare at me there. The books will have large print so that I can learn to read.

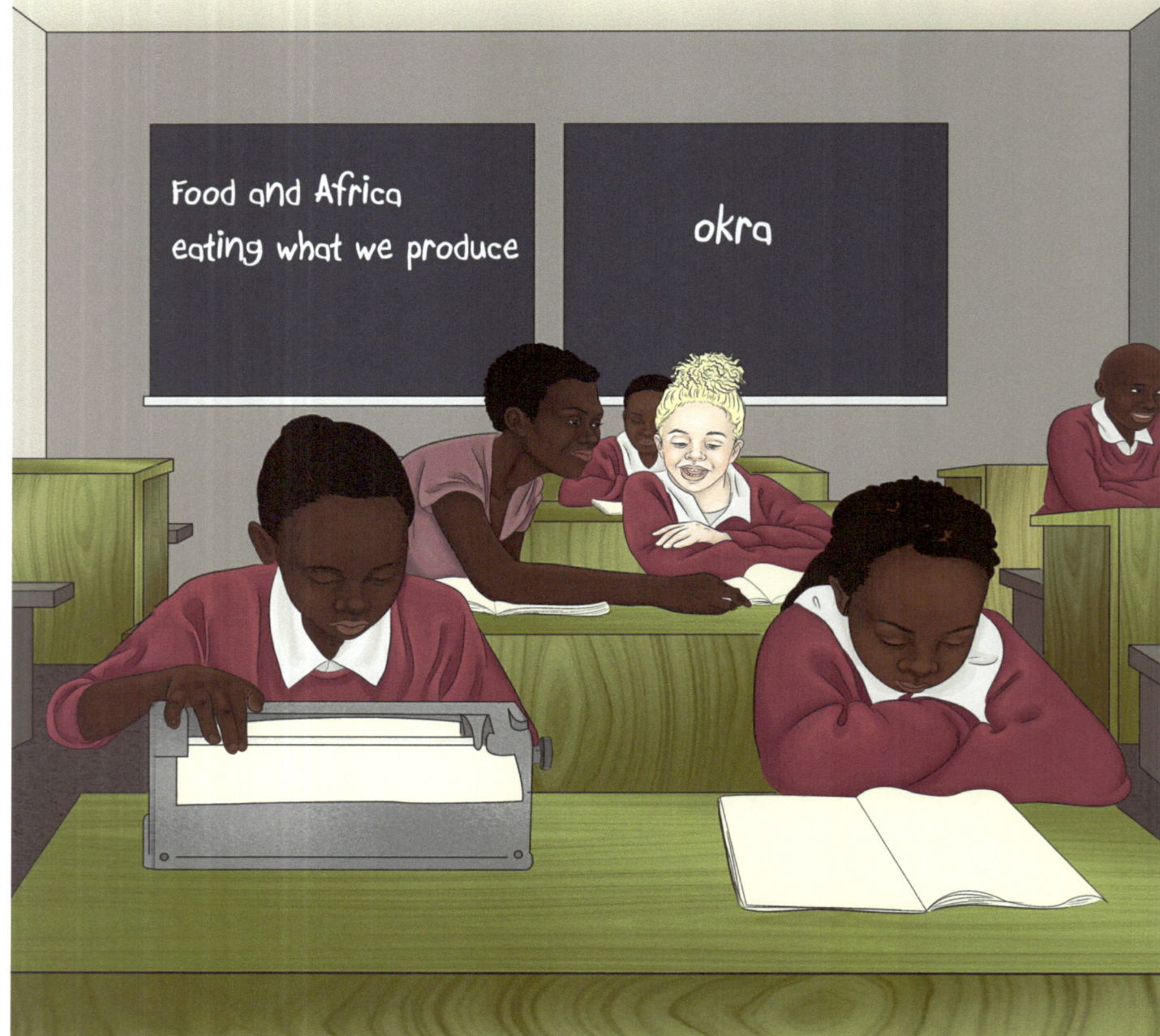

Margaret wonders if I will be afraid to go away to school. I tell her that I have visited the school and everyone is friendly.

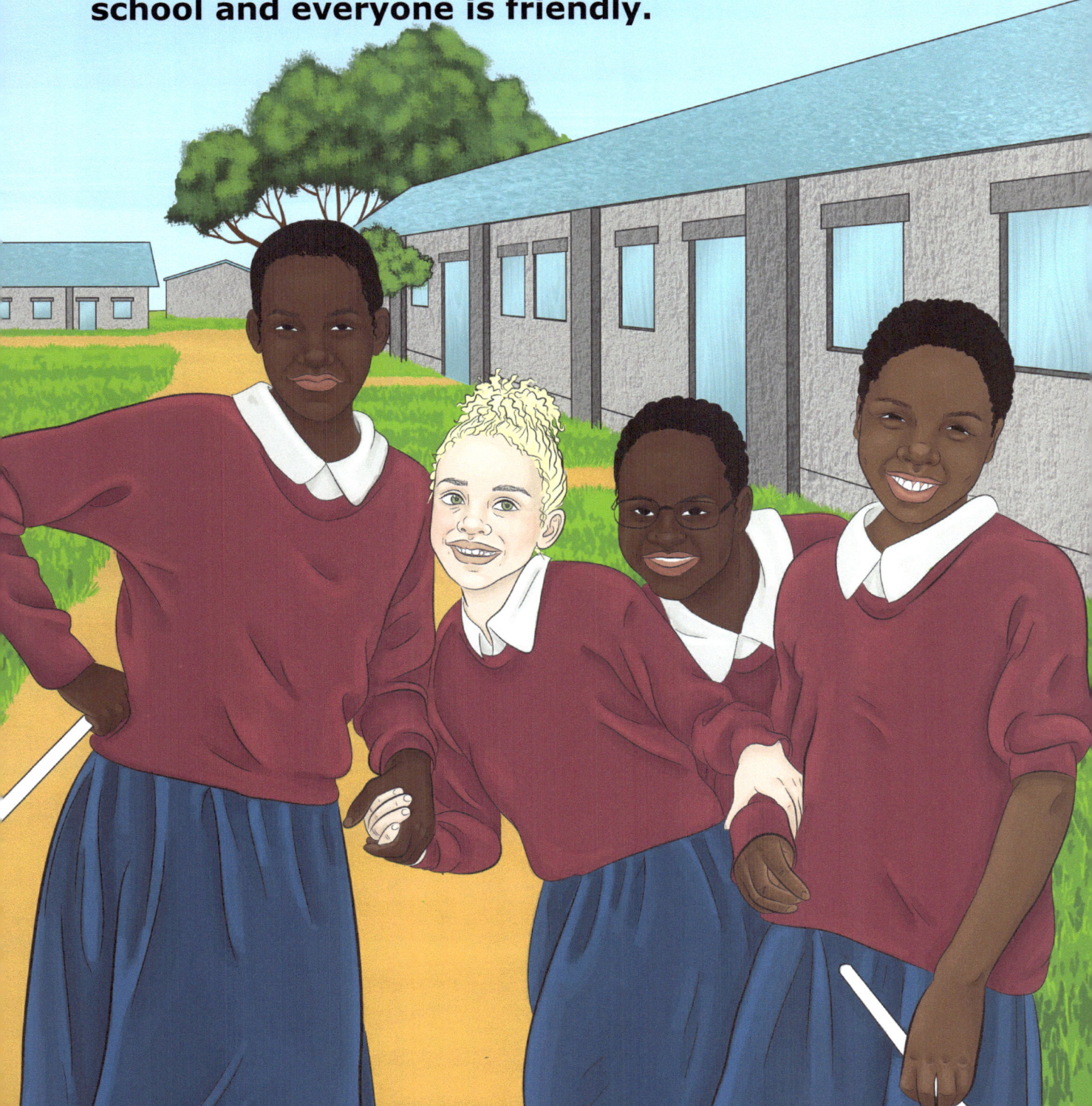

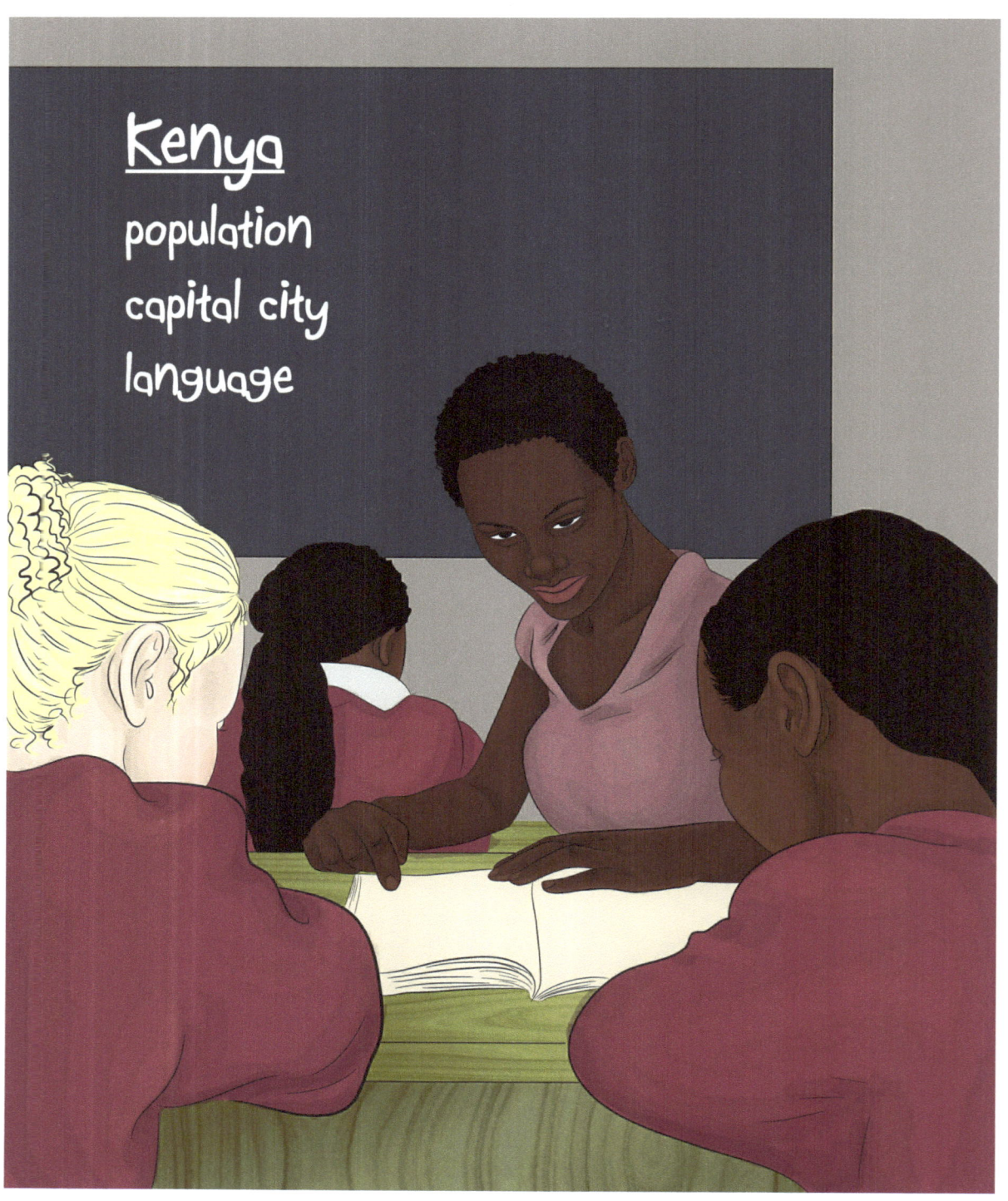

I want to learn how to read and write. This school has books and teachers that can help students like me.

I want to learn to read, do math, and study all the subjects that my older brothers do because I want to be a teacher. I think that Margaret understands because she also wants to learn and become a teacher. And maybe someday, Margaret and I will teach in the same school!

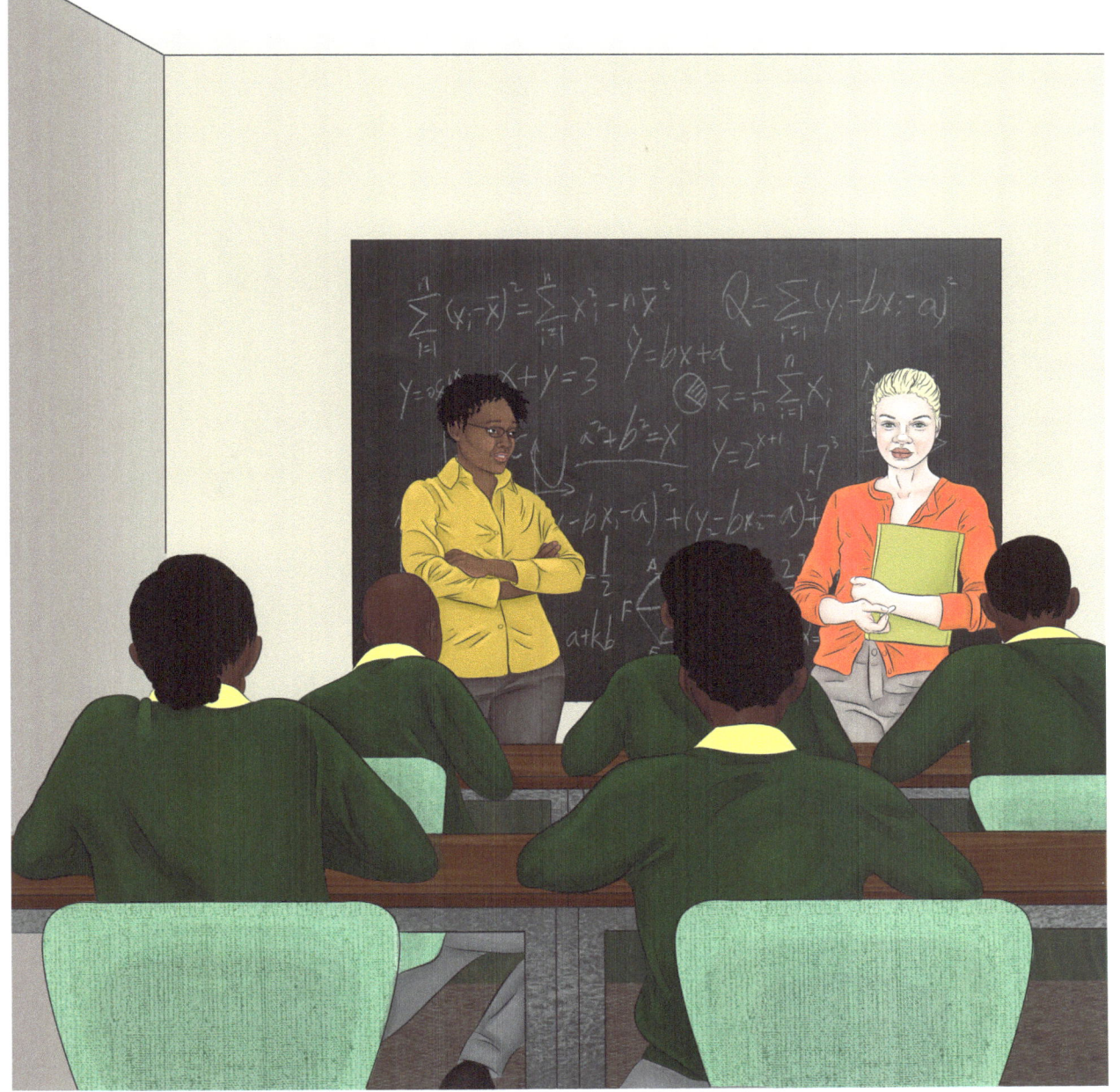

It is time to say goodbye to Margaret. My Mother and I walk home hand in hand and talk about our day at the tea buying center.

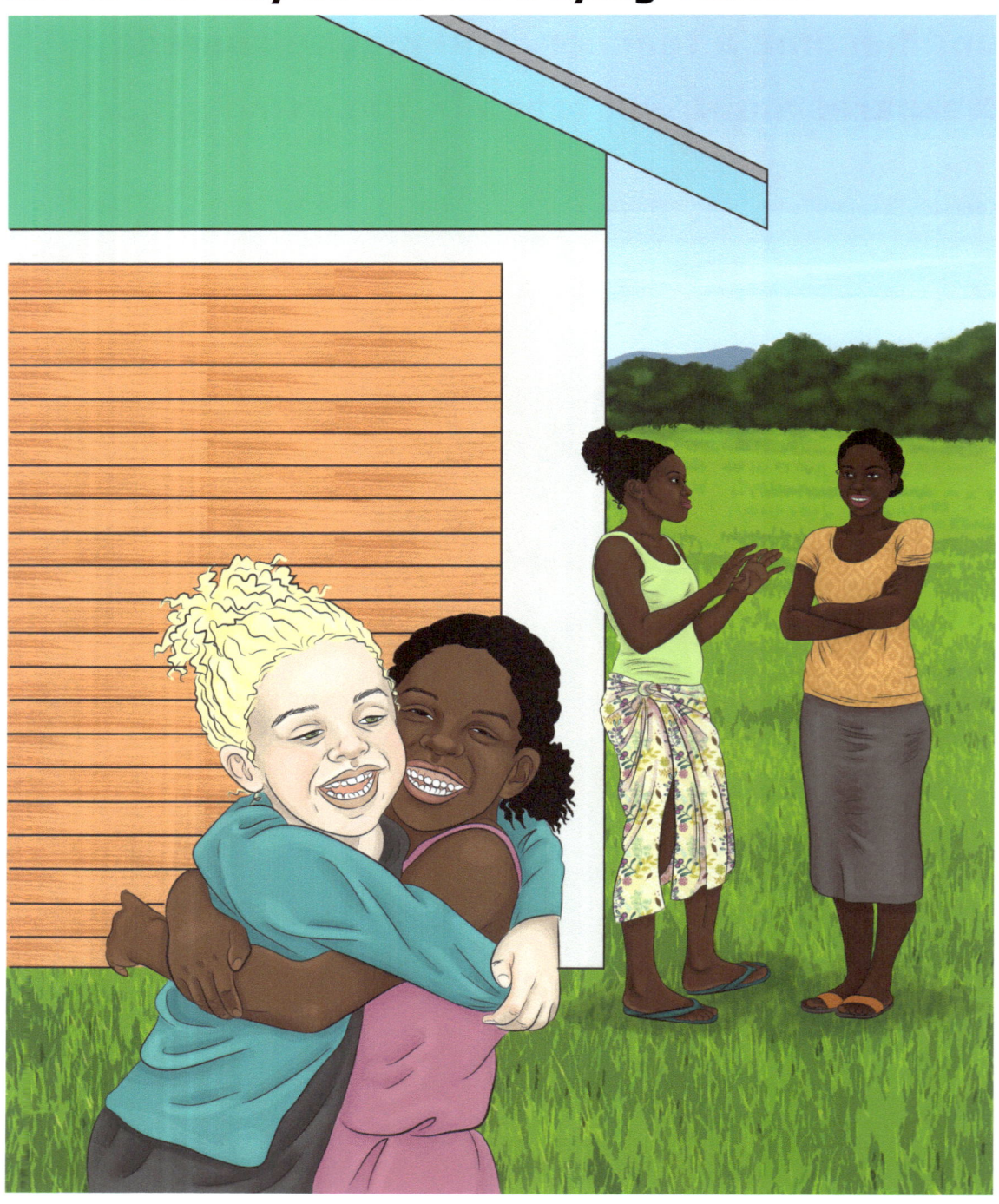

We saw many of our neighbors today and we were able to catch up on the news from many families. I look forward to seeing my friend Margaret next week. Tomorrow I will have time to plant that avocado pit so my family can enjoy avocados at home!

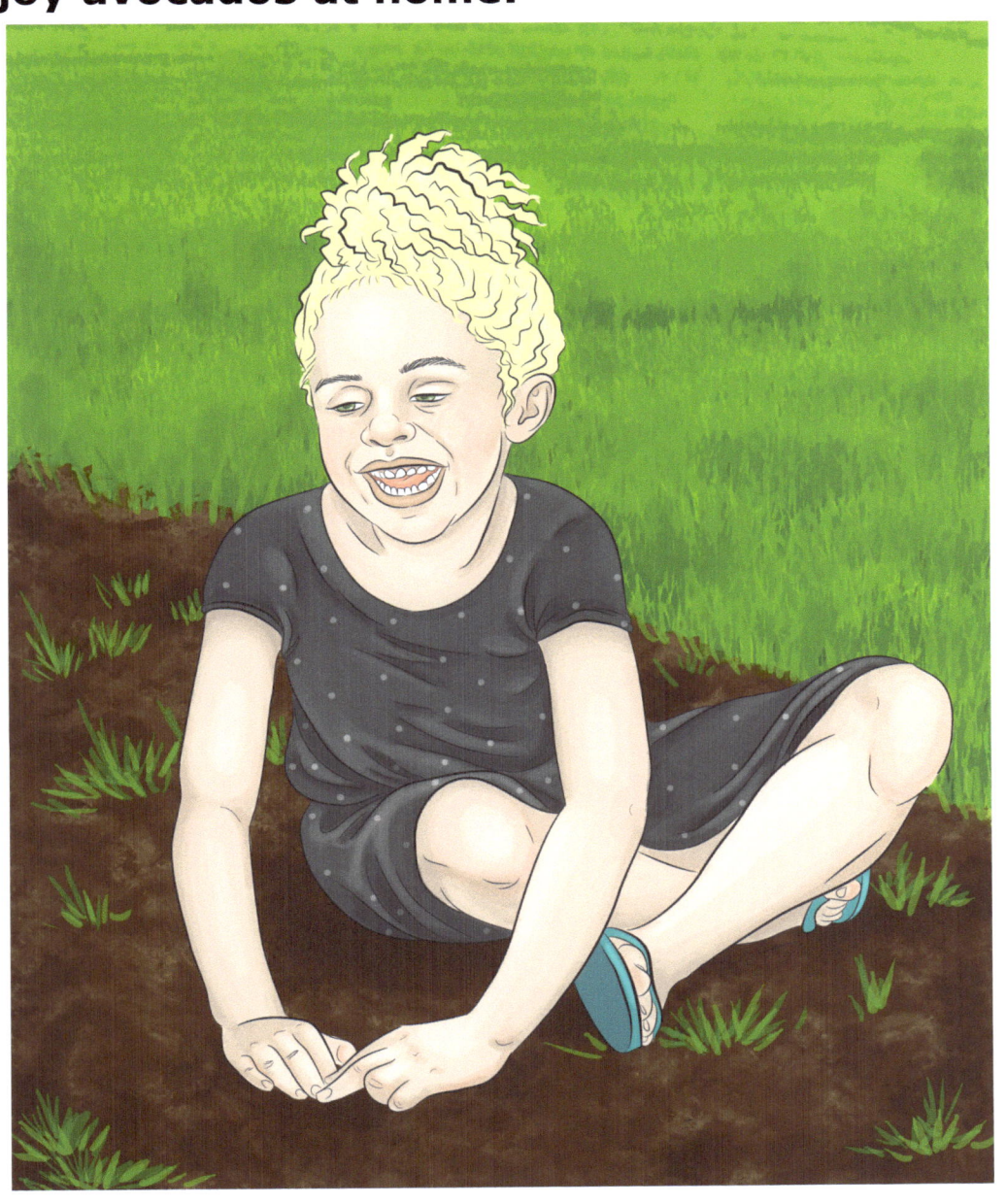

24

About the Authors

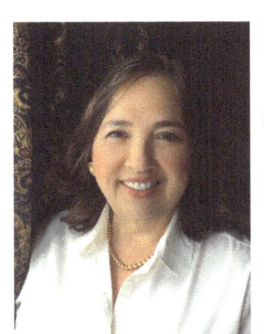

Dr. Sharon Maida has been teaching blind and visually impaired children for 30 years. She has taught braille and is an orientation and mobility specialist in private practice. Sharon is the author of two other books, *Reaching, Crawling, Walking... Let's Get Moving* and *Dynamic Systems Approach to the Development of Creeping*. She is dedicated to improving education for blind children around the world.

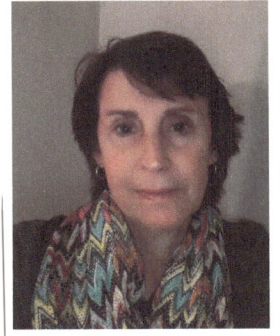

Dr. Lillian Rankel, a research chemist at Mobil, changed careers to become a high school chemistry and physics teacher in 1996. In 2006, she had a blind student in Honors Chemistry who utilized her adaptations and tactile methods to complete the course, including labs. She subsequently co-authored a large print/braille book, *Out-of-Sight Science Experiments*. Dr. Rankel is working to improve education at a blind grammar school in Kenya.

www.ingramcontent.com/pod-product-compliance
Lightning Source LLC
Chambersburg PA
CBHW060810290525
45792CB000053A/1599